Coconut, The Ultimate Superfood: The Benefits Of Coconut Water and Coconut Oil Explained

Table of Contents

Introduction

Coconut water comes from the coastal fruit coconut. Anyone who has been to a coastal area either for business or leisure will come back saying he took coconut or at least saw it. The coconut fruit has a lot of medicinal myths where some are facts and others lie. The most important thing is their medicinal values. This is where the coconut water now comes in with a lot of benefits. The indigenous people of various coastal areas bragged themselves of good health but their secret was later unveiled. They were making use of their naturally available fruit, the coconut.

The coconut water can act as an alternative to water as it has a quenching ability. It is also tasty and carries a lot of nutrients that have a lot of health benefits.

Coconut Water And Weight Loss

The current generation is heavily concerned with issues to do with weight loss. Many doctors always advice their patients to lose weight for a healthy living. With all this pressures many people try very different methods of weight loss. Now, this is where the coconut water comes in.

The coconut has an advantage to human beings as they help in weight loss. It has very little fat contents in them and so a lot of it can be consumed without the fear of getting the pounds of fat in your body. The water also makes you feel full as it suppresses your appetite and this will obviously make you reduce the intake of the other foods.

Coconut Water And The Skin

Almost everyone in this world would do anything for a perfect smooth skin. The coconut water is an answer for this. For those people who have rashes in their skin or any kind of blemish then coconut water is one of the best medicines to go for. This is because it has the ability to tone up the skin and adequately clear them up. The coconut water also moisturizes the skin from within especially if it is taken orally and this advantage can be proved by the products in the market such as the shampoos as one of their ingredients is the coconut water.

The coconut water also prevents the skin from being infected by infections. The skin infections mainly occur during summers or during the monsoons. The coconut water has a lot of healing effect because it contains anti fungal and anti viral properties. One can apply it directly or even mix it with the bathing water. Both processes will be effective and the results will surprise you.

The coconut water is also very advantageous for the oiled skinned people. The coconut oil helps to wash away the excess oil in the skin and keeps the skin tone even. Most people with the oily skin tend to have a shiny face but the coconut water prevents the shine and gives the skin a natural glow.

Coconut Water And Digestion

Coconut water is rich in fiber which is always an important factor during digestion process. If you are always encountering a problem in digestion then coconut water can be a source of relief to you. Because of the high concentration of fiber it will aid in the prevention of indigestion and any occurrence of acid reflux.

Hangovers

Sometimes people over drink and the amount can be so much that the stomach cannot handle it. In drinking too much many of the electrolytes in the stomach will get lost especially through vomiting or constant urination. The coconut water will plat a great role in replacing this water.

Boosts Hydration

Whenever you do any physical exercise, a lot of water is lost in the body. The ingredients in the coconut water are much more effective in hydrating the human body than the sports energy drinks or any of those kinds of drinks. The coconut water acts as a very important form of replacement as it contains natural sugars and potassium in large amounts, unlike the sport drinks and the energy drinks that have very little contents of potassium and the natural sugars. Physical exercise always makes one lose a lot of the mineral rich fluids and the simple replacement of them will be done by the coconut water. Sodium is also an important mineral that is found in the coconut water.

Nutrients In Them

The coconut is absolutely one of the best in terms of the nutrients contents. Obviously many learned people and those who understand issues to deal with a healthy living will go for the best type of drinks to take. This is where many will opt far the coconut drink because it has numerous nutrients in them. The coconut water unlike the other beverages contains a lot of nutrients and the main ones are potassium, sodium, phosphorus, magnesium and calcium. These unique set of nutrients makes it possible for any person with any form of medical condition to enjoy a drink of coconut water.

Blood Pressure

This is a very dangerous condition in the human life. When someone experiences either low or high blood pressure then they are in a very high risk of losing their lives. Statistics show that in the current world many people die because of this condition even more than the very dangerous diseases that you know. The good part is that the condition can be suppressed in many ways but it depends on the type that you are going to use. Taking the coconut water is a very effective way of controlling the condition. In many instances the level of electrolytes in the body can vary and this can lead to high pressure. Coconut water contains a lot of this electrolytes and it ca be used as a means to stabilize the pressure. In many instances, it is recommended that coconut water should be taken at the very start of each day so as to foster the balance of these electrolytes.

Compatibility With Human Blood

The coconut water is isotonic to the human blood. In this case it can be used even in the extreme emergencies to rehydrate the body that is if it administered intravenously.

Aging Factor

Coconut water is also known to be good in keeping you young that is physically young. It contains important elements that are used in the process of cell growth and their regulation. It also has properties that keep the body tissues hydrated and strong for longer and also balances the pH levels.

Kidney Stones

The coconut water helps in the dissolving of the kidney stones mainly because of the presence of potassium which alkalizes preventing the formation of the kidney stones.

Energy Boosting

Coconut water contains a lot of nutrients which makes it a very wonderful energy drink. The water has less sugar and sodium content but high in potassium which makes it possible to replenish the energy.

Increased Metabolic Rate

Coconut water is good in increasing the metabolic rate in humans. Increased metabolic rate is a sign of a healthy person. Regular consumption of the water increases the metabolic rate and this will increase the burn of sugar a lot faster. This will make a person has more energy and hence losing fat more easily.

- Pregnant mothers are very delicate and need to be taken care of with much care. The coconut water is very important to these expectant mothers.

- The coconut water is very good in fighting bacteria especially in the pregnant mothers. It is naturally sterile and helps to improve the immunity of both the mother and the fetus. The anti-bacterial property enables it to prevent infection and illness during the pregnancy.

- The coconut water also gives a very good complexion to the body of the developing child. It is recommended that it should be taken with turmeric for good results.

- Pregnant mothers alas suffer the problem of acidity and they always go for drug in such an event. This should not be the case; instead coconut water should be given to her so as to relieve her from the acidity.

- It is good to note that the coconut water also boosts the fetus health by increasing the amount of amniotic fluid in the womb of the mother.

- Doctor's advice on pregnant women is to go for natural things. This is where the coconut oil comes in as it is natural and contains no artificial flavorings or coloring in them.

- The coconut water also treats infection in the pregnant women, for example it treats the urinary tract and gets rid of infections naturally.

The hair in human beings is the most conspicuous part and every one will do their best to keep them attractive. The coconut oil has adverse importance on the human hair.

- The coconut water fights the issue to do with hair loss in humans. This is because it improves the blood circulation and strengthens the follicles and thus making the hair dense making it looks very attractive.

- The coconut oil also plays an important role in the prevention of dryness in the human hair. The dry and fizzy hair is always hard to manage and therefore there is need too make them moisturized. For it to be easy you need to massage your hair with the coconut water before you bathe and you will get wonderful results.

- The coconut water is also very important in the growth of hair. Its antibacterial properties protect the hair from dandruff and lice which can all hinder hair growth.

- If you are interested in a very shiny hair then the coconut water is very essential in this. It contains vitamins that are essential in maintaining the hair.

- Prevention of the hair breakage is also an important benefit of the coconut oil. This is because it contains a certain acid that give water conditioning abilities. The acids shield the hair proteins and hence protect the root of the hair strand.

Air Circulation

Poor oxygen circulation in the skin leads to impurities in the skin. Every cell in the body requires adequate oxygen supply. This is possible only through proper blood circulation in the body. Coconut water is very important in boosting the air circulation in the body. This will know allow the skin to breathe very healthy air and hence the complexion will improve.

How Much Should You Take?

The coconut oil can be enjoyed when drink alone or can also be enjoyed when you combine with another drink. There are really no guidelines in the amount of coconut water that you should take but it is recommended that you take the water to a certain limit because the water contains a certain amount of calories. A lot of calories in the body are really not that healthy. When you come across different types of coconuts in the market and you are wondering which one to be the best for the water, then don't go for the ones with a hard shell because obviously they are mature and the amount of the water might be less. Instead go for the ones that are still green because they are the ones that have the bet components of the coconut water. Another way to judge the best is to shake the coconut and take the one that has a lot of the water.

In general, the coconut oil is actually one of the best drinks. This is so because of all the advantages mentioned. Always take a good step in your life especially in matters to do with your health and you will be a great person. The coconut fruit is available in almost every country in the world and hence we can say that the water will always available. Don't be left behind and go for it because you will not be discouraged.

Health Benefits Of Coconut Oil

The human body is very delicate and it requires a lot of attention. That is why a lot of research has been done even with the coconut fruit and very important things have been found on the fruit. The fruit contains answers to many health problems of the current world. The fruit is mainly found in the coastal areas or areas near large water mass. One of the products of the fruits is the coconut oil which has adverse advantages to the human being and also the animals. It is quite important for people to learn the importance of some of the fruits in their immediate environment.

Coconut Oil And Weight Loss

Obesity is one of the major concerns of many people in the world. For you to live healthily you need to reduce your weight. Many doctors will always recommend their patients to hit the gym so as to reduce the fat in their body. The coconut oil is found to increase the amount of energy used in the body and hence burning fatter in your body. Then if you think you are overweight then don't hesitate to try it and be pretty sure of great results.

Birth Marks And Age Spots

It is almost certain that almost everyone has birth marks. These are the marks that we just don't get them when we play out there with our friends when we were young but those that we are born with. Some people think that they are permanently there.

The age marks are also got when someone becomes old. The coconut oil has a property that makes it able to erase these marks. In the age marks you need to apply it directly to the spot. Supplement the coconut oil with the laser removal treatment for effective removal. The oil can also be used to remove the stretch marks. Some of the people who have already lost some of their weight now have the problem with the stretch marks. But it's simple, just apply the oil and you will be amazed with the results.

Baldness

Baldness can be normal to some people and they can appreciate the way they are without worrying about anything. To some others this is a real problem and hence they will look for ways that they can make their hair grow. You can apply the coconut oil to the affected areas three times a day because the oil supports cell regeneration.

The coconut oil can also be used as an after shave. Don't be stressed by the pimples that reoccur immediately after you shave. The coconut oil will clean your skin after shaving without clogging the pores.

Body Scrub

The coconut oil can also be used as an effective body scrub. Mix the coconut oil with sugar and scrub tour body. Many people have the belief that if your body becomes smooth then you become more attractive. You can try this oil and you will be sure of a smooth skin. You can later apply any other oil depending on your choice of the smell.

Bruises And Burns

Sometimes we are accidentally cut by something or even by other people. Don't be stressed of your bruise or burn will heal. Try and apply the oil to the bruise and be amazed. The coconut oil increases the rate of healing by reducing the redness and the swelling. Also apply to the part where you have been burnt and continue adding until when it is healed. The oil will reduce the chances of permanent marks appearing in the body and it promotes healing. Also sometimes you can be bite by a bug. Don't rush to a clinic or something of that sort. Just relax and apply the coconut oil because it will reduce the itching and hasten the healing process.

Dandruff Remover And Eye Creamer

The coconut oil is very good in removing the dandruffs which are mostly located in the head. Dandruffs are mostly due to the dryness of the skin. The oil moisturizes the dry skin and hence reduces the symptoms of dandruffs. Oil secretion from the skin is also another cause of dandruffs and so the oil will control the oil secretion from the scalp. The oil can also be used as an eye creamer. Apply the oil to prevent wrinkling. Use on the lids mostly in the evening.

Face Wash And Hair Treatment

Sometimes negate the use of the normal soap and try another different alternative to even bigger results. Mix the coconut oil with olive oil. Try one tablespoonful of the oil. Wet the face first then rub the oil. Leave for some few minutes then wash it. To apply it in your head, take a tablespoonful and rub it all over your head. Cover your head so that it does not make the beddings dirty. Leave overnight and then wash your head the first thing in the morning.

Lubricant And Make Up Remover

- The coconut oil can also be used as lubricant as it naturally self person lubricant but it is not compatible with latex. It is also amazing that the coconut oil can remove the make your in your skin. Just use a piece of cotton and a small amount of coconut oil and see how amazing it works. The oil can also be used as massage oil. This is a very simple process you just grab some and scrub it on the body.

- The oil can also be used as a moisturizer and it's so simple because you just scoop some of it and you rub it all over your body, including the neck

- Coconut oil can also be used as safe cooking oil especially for deep frying. Deep fried food is not always recommended by the doctors because of the huge amounts of fats in them. The coconut oil is not like the normal oil and hence it is very good in deep frying.

- The coconut oil can also be applied immediately after doing the dishes so as to avoid dry skin. The babies can also use the oil because it is a natural baby lotion.

- The oil can also be used to kill yeast and yeast infections. They also are useful in support healthy thyroid function.

Benefits Of Coconut Oil In Dogs

A dog is a very important animal in the human life. Many people have kept the animals pet just for fun while others for work, for example for security. Then, the animal needs to be really taken care of. The coconut oil is also a very important substance in the dog's life.

- First, the coconut oil improves the overall skin health of the dog and prevents the dog from being infected by any type of infections.

- The oil also plays an important role in moisturizing the skin of the dog. This is whether you apply it orally or even mix it with a shampoo.

- Applied directly to the skin of the dog, the oil heals the dog from the wound or any type of cuts that the dog might have.

- Many dogs have a really bad odor. But this should not worry you because the coconut oil can overcome that. The antibacterial property of the coconut oil and its sweet tropical aroma will give your dog a very pleasant smell.

- The coconut oil also prevents yeast infections. The yeast infections are the ones that are responsible for many dog diseases. The antiviral agents in the oil also make the dog recover faster especially from the kennel cough.

- Dogs also have many stomach problems and one of them is digestion and also nutrient absorption. Don't leave your dog to suffer from indigestion or problems related to that and you are just be sited there thinking that all is well because the dog is an animal. It also has its rights! Add the coconut oil to the dog's diet. If the stool of the dog becomes lose then its simple just give it a canned pumpkin.

- Some dogs are overweight and they need proper health assistance if they are going to reduce to a manageable level. You need not to look for a better alternative; the coconut oil can be the best choice for you. Research also shows that dogs with some smell from their mouth can benefits from this oil. You need not to take that extra chance and brush your dog's teeth when you can employ this oil.

- Coconut oil has also been beneficial in dealing and coping with diabetes. This capability can be achieved because this oil regulates, maintains and checks on the amount of insulin in the body. It has also been found to reduce the risk of heart diseases. In addition to this, it improves the functioning on the thyroid.

- Dogs like humans suffer from memory loss. If you are looking for the best medicine that will be less costly and natural then you need to use the coconut oil. This will make them energetic, alert and strong irrespective of their age.

The benefits of coconut oil are not only numerous but also wide. They find use both in humans and in the animal kingdom. All you need to do is to find the perfect use that will suit your situation, keep you healthy and strong all the time.

www.ingramcontent.com/pod-product-compliance
Lightning Source LLC
Chambersburg PA
CBHW060107300526
45787CB00018B/1856